Understanding the Alexander Technique

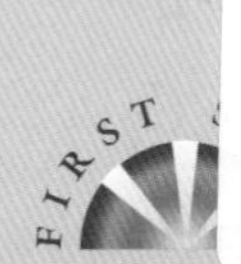

Contents

1 Understanding the Therapy 4

Who invented it?; Who can it help?; Working together.

2 A Brief History 8

Early childhood; The performer; Primary control; Bound for Britain; In practice; The legacy.

3 How It Works? 16

Finding the balance; Applying the principle; The connection; Modern man.

4 The Magic Formula 24

The thought process; Putting it together.

5 Teaching The Alexander Technique 32

Blocks to learning; Moment of inhibition; State of communion; The harmonic principle; Thinking together; Leading from within; The wider application.

6 Will The Alexander Technique Work For Me? 44

Structural conditions; Nervous conditions; High performance; What will I learn? How long will it take?

7 Three Great Benefits 52

Pain management; Finding pleasure; The radiant way.

8 How To Find Us 61

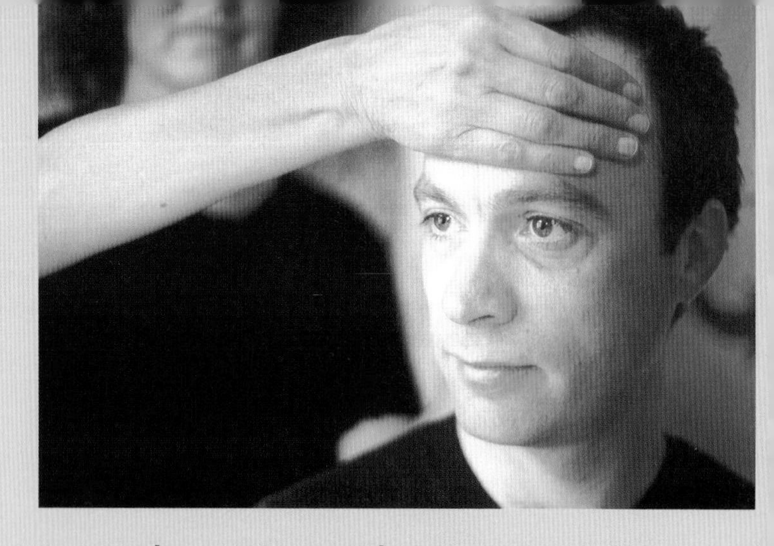

1 Understanding The Therapy

The Alexander Technique offers a completely different approach to other body work therapies, in that you, the 'pupil', become aware with the 'teacher' of how to think into your body.

Together, using Alexander principles, you will learn to re-evaluate the relationship between your mind and your body.

WHO INVENTED IT?

The technique is named after Frederick Matthias Alexander, an Australian actor, who started to experience voice difficulties which doctors failed to diagnose. Through a process of self-observation, using three mirrors, Alexander discovered that the condition was caused by a faulty relationship between the head to the neck, and the neck to the back.

He found out that the effects of this breakdown in balance are far-reaching, leading to many of the chronic conditions suffered in the modern world.

WHO CAN IT HELP?

The Alexander Technique can be used to help many different people, but basically its application falls into three main spheres.

- It helps to enhance performance. If you are an actor, a singer, a musician, or an athlete, the Alexander Technique will be a positive aid, as well as helping you to avoid many of the physical injuries caused by over-use of one part of the body.

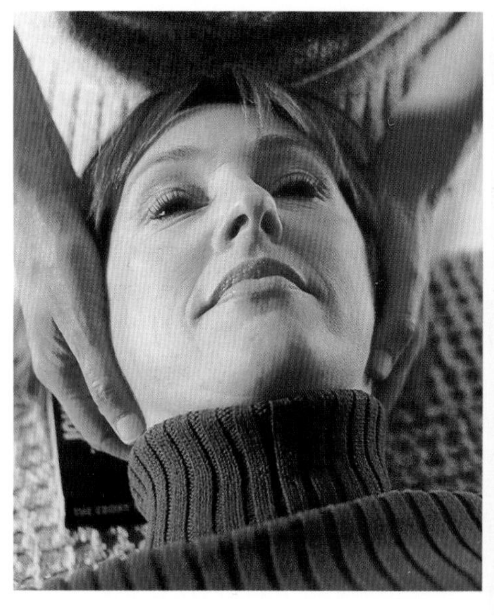

▲ *The pupil must learn to work with the teacher.*

- It is of enormous help to those suffering from long-term back problems, frozen shoulders, recurring stiff necks and migraines. People who suffer from breathing problems and asthmatic conditions have also received great benefits.

- Finally, the Alexander Technique can help people to cope with pain, and can be beneficial to those who have stress-related problems.

WORKING TOGETHER

The Alexander Technique requires the active participation of the 'pupil', who must learn to work with the teacher. The mind must be totally involved and engaged in order to get results.

Like most things that are worthwhile, it takes time to get the full benefits from the Alexander Technique – and the longer you practise it, the greater your rewards will be.

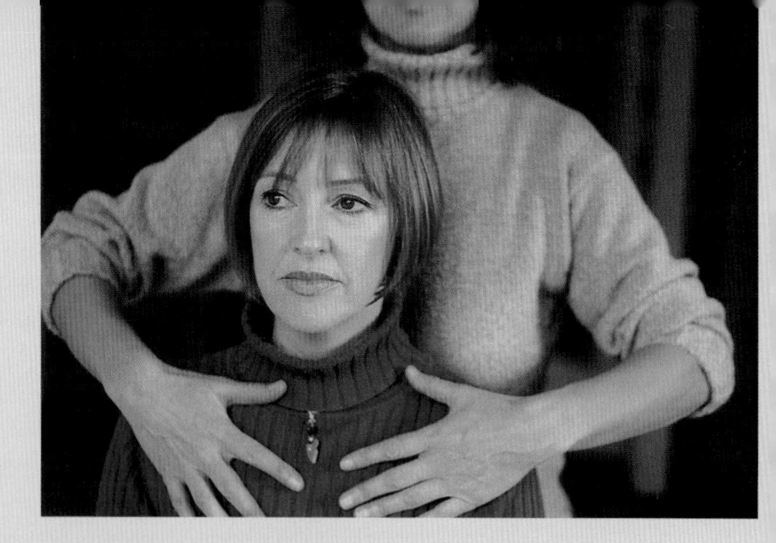

2 A Brief History

Frederick Matthias Alexander was born in Tasmania in 1869. He was a sickly child, which kept him in the position of the quiet observer of his large family.

EARLY CHILDHOOD

His mother was a midwife and rode to her work on horseback. One of Alexander's earliest memories was of his mother, rushing to a birth, jumping over the gate on her horse – and the horse's neck lengthening beautifully as it sailed over the gate.

Because of his poor health, Alexander was educated at home. He was a thoughtful child and liked to ask his tutor difficult questions, such as "How do you know what you know?"

This early respect for real knowledge, based on original thought and experience, was to be the foundation of his discoveries later on in life.

THE PERFORMER

When his father died, Alexander became the head of the family. He went to work in the offices of the mining companies, travelling widely and mixing with lots of different people.

However, this did not deflect him from his great ambition to become an actor, and to recite Shakespeare in front of an audience.

Eventually, Alexander realised his dream, and became well-known for his Shakespearean recitations. But then disaster struck: Alexander started to lose his voice.

He tried every cure he could find, but no one could diagnose the cause of the problem, or alleviate his suffering.

At this point in the story, most people would give up and go back to the old 'day job' – not the young pioneer from Tasmania.

He embarked on a journey of self-discovery, determined to find the cause of his problem.

His one guiding principle was that he knew that it was something that he was doing to himself that caused him to lose his voice.

PRIMARY CONTROL

For the next few years, Alexander observed himself with the help of three mirrors. As a result of his observations, he came up with a profound discovery.

He uncovered a principle in nature that is shared by all vertebrates (all creatures that have spines) from snakes to horses, to man. He called this principle the primary control.

It is based on the relationship between the head, the neck and the back, which, according to Alexander, affects the entire co-ordination of the rest of the body. He believed it involved the mental processes, enabling the body to revitalise itself.

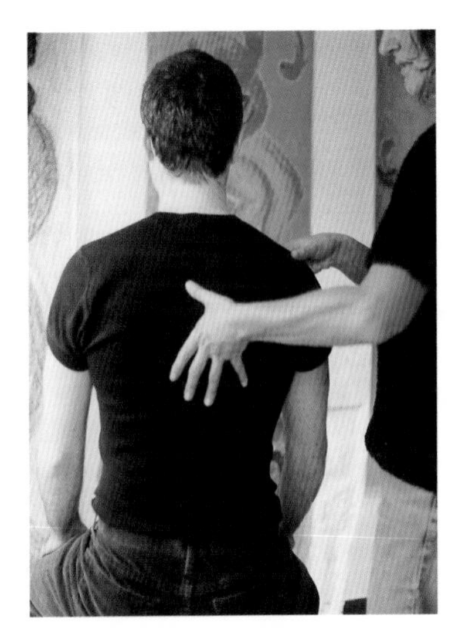

▲ *The primary control: The relationship between the head, the neck and the back.*

Alexander used this principle on himself, and soon his voice was restored. News of this startling 'cure' spread, and Alexander was called in to help other actors who had voice and breathing difficulties.

BOUND FOR BRITAIN

News travels fast in the theatrical world, and in 1905 the great playwright George Bernard Shaw invited Alexander to come to Britain to promote his new technique.

The only problem was finding the fare. Here, the other side of his life came in handy. Alexander had always had a good eye for a horse, so he headed straight for the race track. A bet on a horse with a strong neck – and the ability to lengthen at the crucial last stretch – did the trick.

Soon Alexander was heading for London, and while he was making the long voyage from Australia to England, he started writing a book about his new discovery.

In London, he was welcomed by the leading intellectuals of the day: Bernard Shaw, Stafford

Cripps, and later Aldous Huxley and John Dewey, the American educator, became interested in his work.

IN PRACTICE

Alexander set up in practice in London, and soon clients were coming from all walks of life.

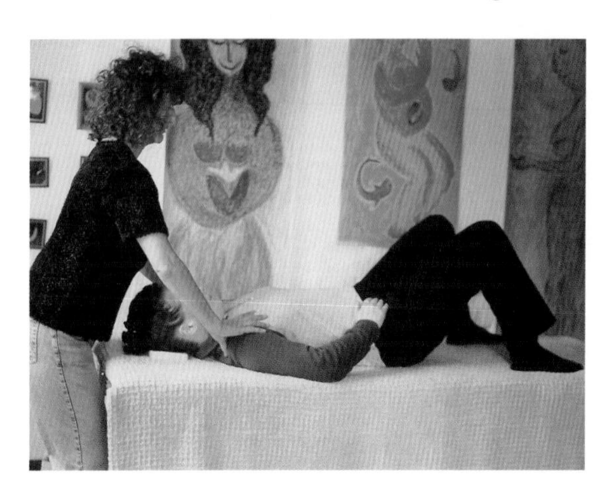

◀ *Soon, Alexander was treating a wide range of patients with many different complaints.*

Initially, he worked with actors, helping them just before they went on stage. He became known as the 'doctor of the London theatre', famous for the results he achieved, working with his hands and his voice.

Later, he became known for treating 'incurables' – the patients everyone else had given up on. From the doctor's son born with a hunched back, to the polio victim, Alexander was able to help them all to help themselves.

Over the years, Alexander founded a school for children, and he also started to train adults who would be able to carry on his work.

With great passion and dedication, Alexander continued to promote his technique until he was in his eighties. He gave up work just a few weeks before he died.

THE LEGACY

Today, the Alexander Technique is widely recognised as a mainstream therapy.

- There are training schools worldwide. The Alexander

Technique is an essential part of the curriculum in many drama and music colleges.

- The therapy is available in most alternative and complementary clinics, as well as being taught privately.
- There is an Alexander Technique Society, with an international membership of practitioners.
- There are books and videos, which give newcomers and practitioners an insight into the technique.

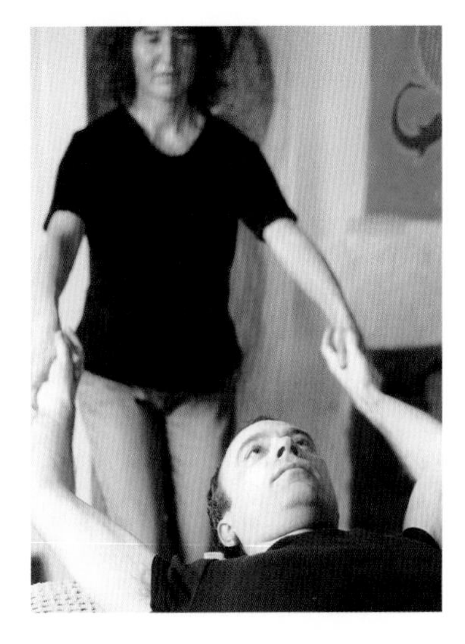

▲ *The Alexander Technique has thrown new light on the relationship between the mind and the body.*

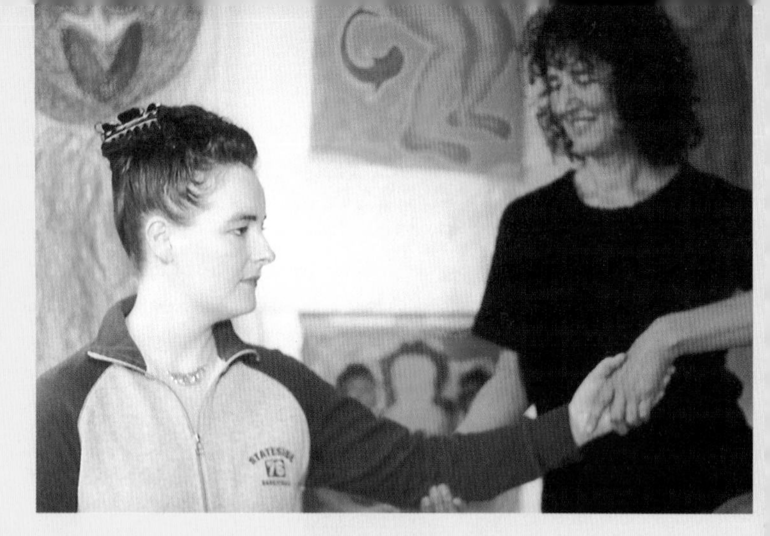

3 How It Works

In order to understand the Alexander Technique, we need to go back to the point in Alexander's life when he was observing himself with three mirrors in the hope of finding a cure for his vocal problems.

FINDING THE BALANCE

Alexander noticed that while he was reciting a speech, he was pulling his head back and down, and tightening his throat.

He then discovered that, although he could not change the use of his throat directly, he could change the relationship of his head to his neck, and this did have an effect on his throat.

He saw that if his head balanced on his neck in such a way as to go forward and up, then the whole of the rest of his spine was able to lengthen.

This, he realised, was the key – the head, neck, back relationship. If that relationship was in order, then many, many other things would follow, such as voice, breathing, tension, and general co-ordination.

Alexander saw this as a primary reflex in man, and he referred to it as the 'primary control'.

Since man is a vertebrate, it was logical to assume that the head, neck, back relationship must apply to all other vertebrates, who would share the same dynamic principles of movement and co-ordination.

All vertebrates would therefore respond to primary control, which was, in fact, a principle of nature that included man.

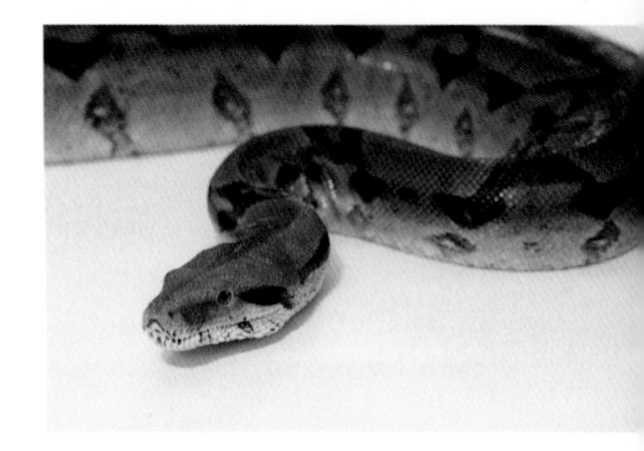

▲ *The head of the snake leads him into movement.*

APPLYING THE PRINCIPLE

To test the principle of primary control, take the simplest of vertebrates, the snake. The head of the snake leads him into movement and his spine follows.

Go one step further and consider a lizard. The head of the lizard leads him into movement, the spine follows and the limbs facilitate, but don't lead.

Take a bird on the wing. The head leads, the spine follows and the wings facilitate the flight.

Take a horse leaping over a fence. The head leads, the spine follows and the limbs facilitate the jump.

Take a small and curious

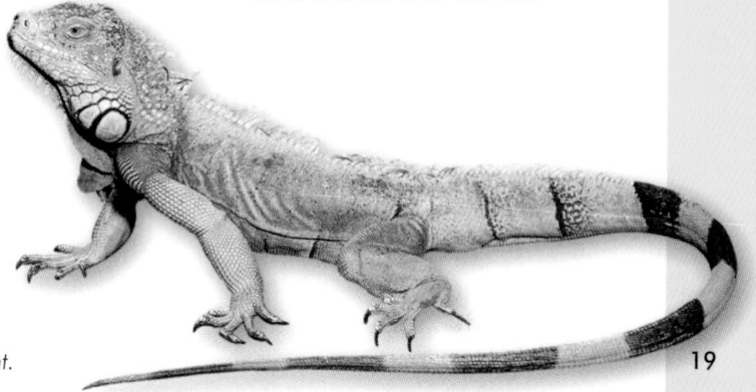

► *When the lizard moves, he is led in to movement by his head, his spine follows, and the limbs facilitate the movement.*

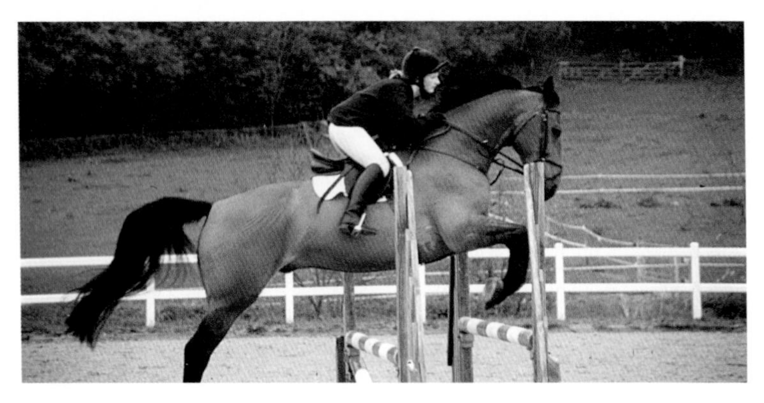

▲ *The horse clears a fence, leading with his head.*

toddler, just learning to walk. The head leads, the spine follows, and the legs facilitate and so do the arms.

Now take the ordinary man in the street at rush hour. The head is falling back and down, the spine is shortening, and the limbs are pushing him onwards – a sorry sight.

THE CONNECTION

Alexander saw his work as reconnecting man to nature, returning to the principles of co-ordination that he shares with all other vertebrates. He wanted man to recapture the grace he once had as a small child, but this time it would have to be through his consciousness, it would have to be a matter of choice.

Alexander had discovered the principle of the primary control, the first reflex, shared by all vertebrates, but he had to find a way of applying the principle.

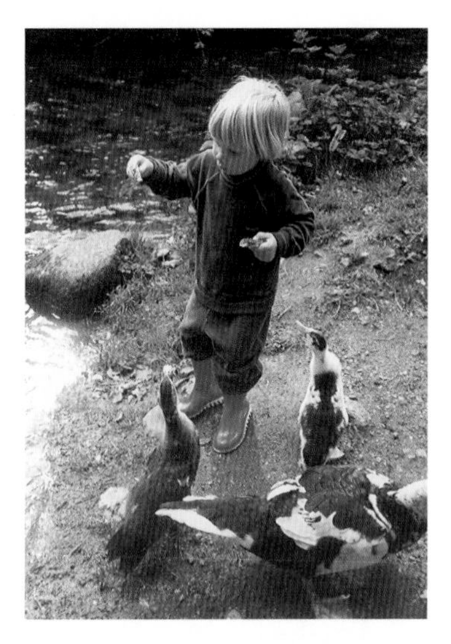

▲ *The curious toddler leads with the head, the spine follows, helped by the legs and arms.*

He needed to find a formula so that ordinary people would be able to restore their basic co-ordination, their original poise, the balance of the head to the neck and to the back.

He was finally able to do this by understanding where modern man had gone wrong – by finding out what caused him to fall from grace.

MODERN MAN

Looking back at history, Alexander saw that, ever since the industrial revolution, both

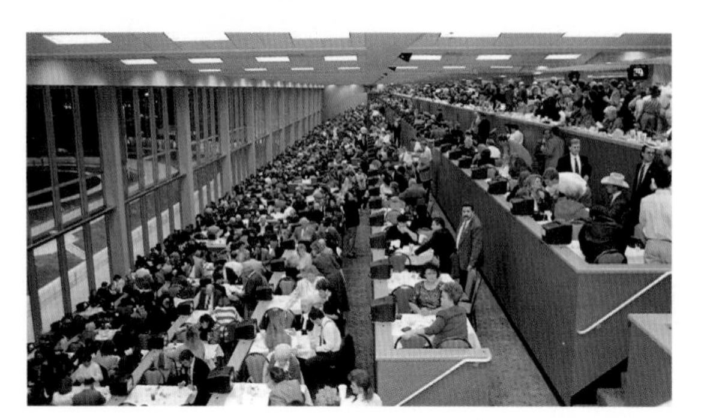

◄ *Post-industrial man has lost his natural sense of balance.*

in farming and in factories, man had been used as a kind of machine.

He no longer did a variety of tasks, or was allowed to rest when he was tired. Modern man had to repeat and repeat the same action, for hours on end, often well past the point of exhaustion.

The constant pressure of repetition, the bracing and fixing against exhaustion, kept man in a shocked state – a state of compression and tension.

The shock reflex is set up in the body to protect it from sudden blows.

- The neck stiffens, it then pulls the head back and down.
- The shoulders raise up and pull in.
- The back narrows and compresses.
- The spine shortens.
- The legs retreat into the hips.

It protects the person, yes, but it is no way to live.

Alexander believed that modern, post-industrial man was, to some extent, living in the shock reflex each and every day of his rushed and repetitive life.

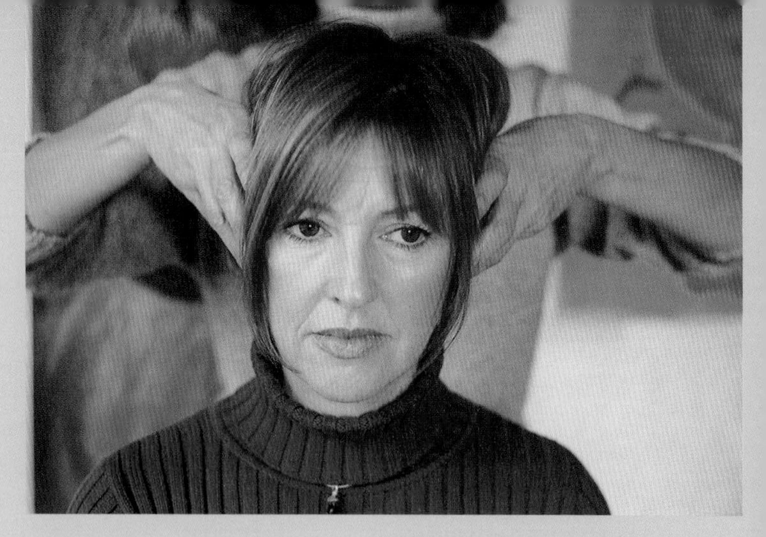

4 The Magic Formula

In order to come out of the shock reflex and restore the good use of the primary control, Alexander developed a series of inter-connected thoughts, or directions, for the body.

Much like 'the house that Jack built', these thoughts build one upon the other until, finally, the whole is created, and can be sustained.

THE THOUGHT PROCESS

- The first thought was to unstiffen the neck, held tight in the shock reflex; to let the neck be free.

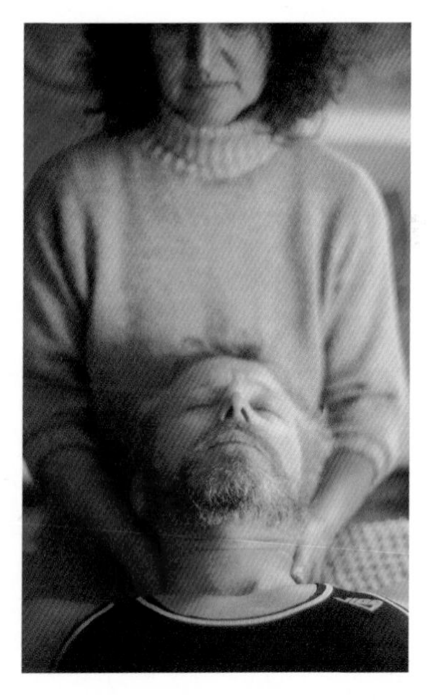

▲ *"Let the neck be free."*

- If the neck was held tightly, it would pull the head back and down, and shorten the spine. Conversely, if the neck was allowed to be free, if it softened and unstiffened, then the head would be free to go forward and up. It would not be pulled back and down.

And so the first two thoughts: *"Let the neck be free"* in order that you can then *"let the head go forward and up"*, comprise the first two directions of Alexander's magic formula.

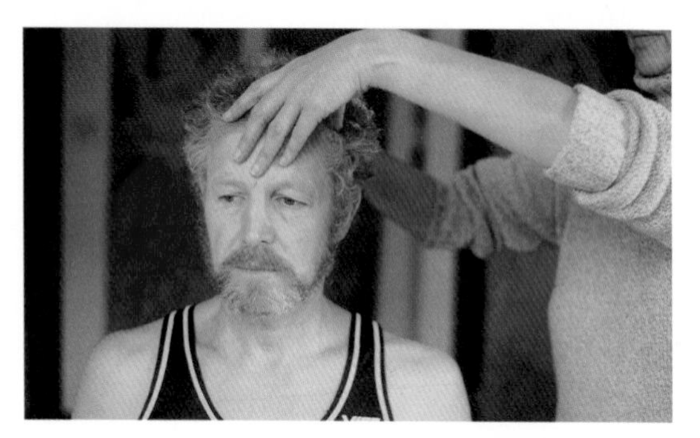

◀ *"The head may go forward and up."*

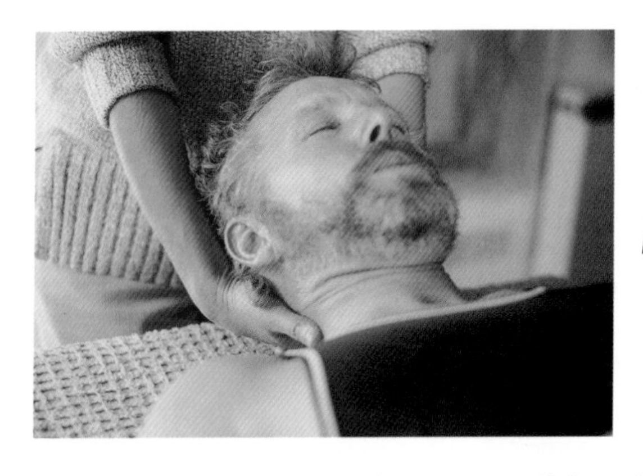

◀ *"The back may lengthen and widen."*

- If the head is going forward and up, it is not shortening the spine. It is, in fact, creating the space and the opportunity for the spine to lengthen – all the way along itself, from the top of the neck to the bottom of the tail.

- If the spine is lengthening, the back itself will have space to widen and open.

So, all around the hips and the ribcage, in a lengthening spine, there is the possibility for the back to widen.

This, in short, is Alexander's solution, his magic formula, to get us out of the shock reflex: *"Let the neck be free, so that the head can go forward and up, so that the back can lengthen and widen."*

Like the house that Jack built, once these three thoughts or directions are working clearly, the structure begins to open, to decompress, and to be organised around the primary control – the head, neck, back relationship.

Alexander continued his thoughts to release the arms and legs from their contraction in the shock reflex.

- To prevent the arms from pulling back and into the shoulders in shock, Alexander gave the directions: *"Out and away across the upper arms"*.

► *Opposite: "Out and away across the upper arms."*

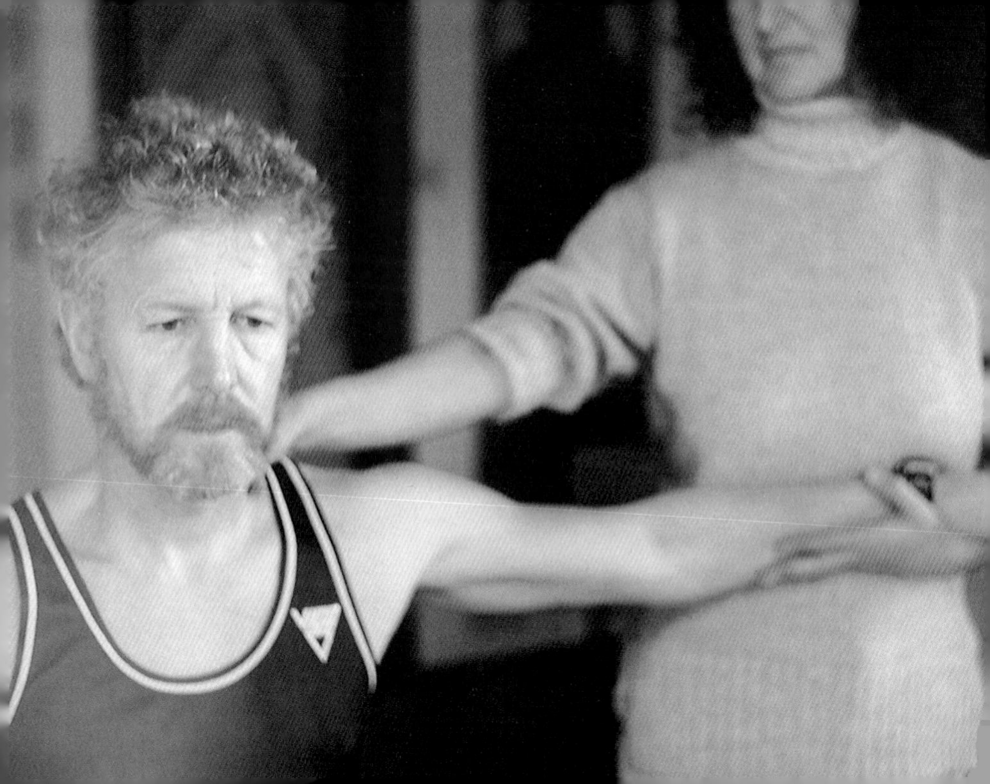

- To prevent the legs pulling backward and inwards into the hips in shock, he gave the direction:
  "Knees forwards and away".

PUTTING IT TOGETHER

If all these instructions or 'thoughts' are put together, you have the entire magic formula of Alexander's

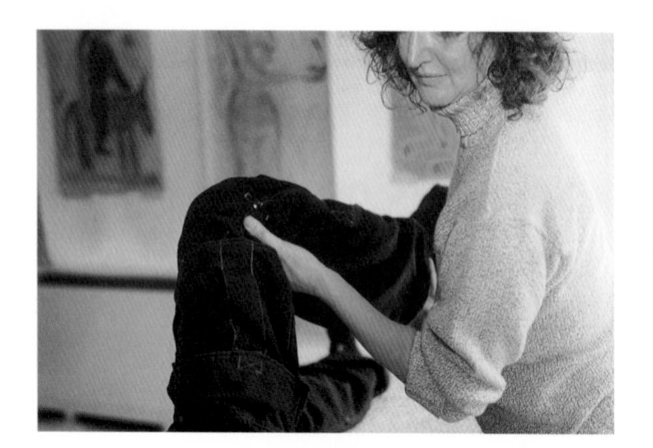

◄ *"Knees forwards and away."*

directions to open the structure, to keep it open, and to prevent it falling into the compression of the shock reflex. It is repeated like a prayer or mantra by the students and teachers of Alexander's technique alike.

> *Let the neck be free, so that the head may go forward and up, so that the back may lengthen and widen. Out and away across the upper arms. Knees forwards and away.*

If it was truly that simple, we would all be able to do it, just like that. This is not the case. In fact, teaching the magic formula is the most complex part of the story.

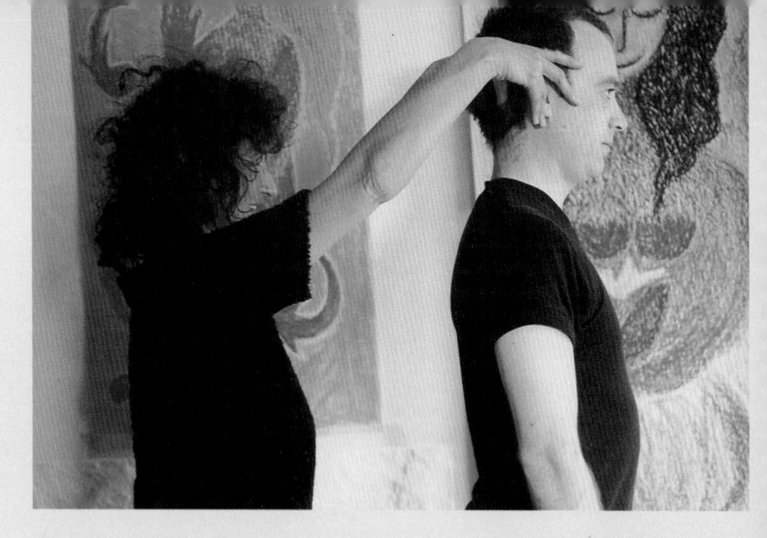

5 Teaching The Alexander Technique

Going from one state of being to another can never be a simple journey. So, unsurprisingly, getting yourself out of the shock reflex – a state of tension under pressure – into a state of harmony with nature, is no easy task. So how did Alexander do it?

BLOCKS TO LEARNING

Observation was the first step of his journey. Alexander observed that when he gave a recitation, he pulled his head back and down, and compressed his throat. He went on to see many other instances of human beings pulling themselves down. How could he effect a change?

At first, Alexander tried putting himself right, by physically making his head go in the correct position on top of his neck, going forward and up.

But then he discovered that he was using the same amount of physical effort as he was in pulling his head back and down. He was simply moving his tension from one place to another. The tension was still with him.

Likewise, in the early stages of teaching, Alexander would see what was wrong with the pupil, and would then shout instructions to them.

But all this achieved was moving the level of stress from one posture to another. It seemed hopeless. And then Alexander discovered the use of the gap, the pause, the brief moment of 'inhibition'.

MOMENT OF INHIBITION

Between stimulus and response, there is a pause. Alexander called this 'inhibition', meaning that moment in the nervous system between stimulus (the telephone ringing, for example) and response (jumping up to answer it).

In this brief pause, Alexander had time to reorganise himself, rather than simply to react in his usual, tense, strained manner. He learned to say no, to wait, and to give his directions for the primary control:

"Neck free, head forward and up..."

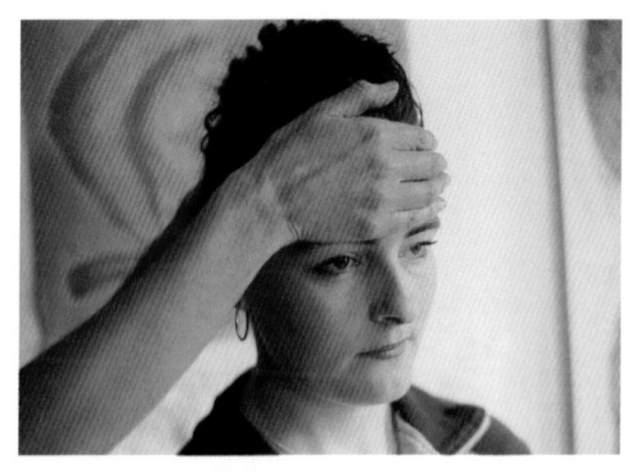

◀ *Between stimulus and response there is a pause – the moment of inhibition.*

As he paused and gave his directions, he noticed that another system, based only on his own strong, positive thinking, kicked into action.

This system was not based on physical exertion; it was a state of non-doing, of pure thinking.

As Alexander paused for this system of non-doing to take over, the whole quality of his muscle tone changed, and when he came to move, he found he was moving with the minimum of effort.

He was coming from somewhere else entirely – namely, the primary control.

STATE OF COMMUNION

Alexander discovered that this state of non-doing could be shared with his pupils if the following pre-requisites were observed.

- Alexander would put his hands on the pupil, for example, at the back of the head and under the jaw, to correct pulling the head back and down.

- At this point, he had to be in the non-doing state of the primary control.

- Using his voice, he would convey himself clearly to set up a system of non-doing with the pupil so they were thinking together.

By using his voice, the pupil was able to listen and join in the thought process, and

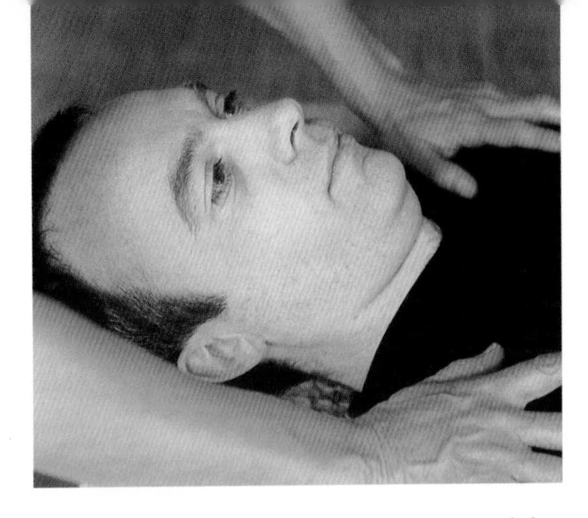

◀ *The teacher has the ability to lead, and the pupil will follow.*

because Alexander was more experienced, the pupil had something to follow.

In other words, Alexander made his body and mind into a state of being first, and then invited the pupil to join him.

Alexander discovered that, if he made himself into the correct environment, if he led by being, then the student could follow. That is, if the

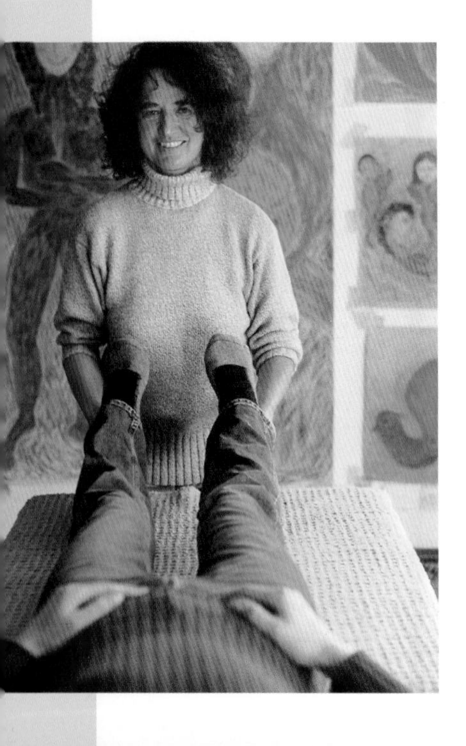

clear thinking instructions were shared.

Thus, Alexander discovered what is known as the 'harmonic principle' for his teaching.

THE HARMONIC PRINCIPLE

Like all the best discoveries, the harmonic principle is extremely simple and, as a result, its application is far-reaching.

- If you stand next to a good singer in a choir, and you

◀ *Freeing the legs in the hips. The directions for primary control are learnt in relative stillness.*

yourself are not particularly good at holding a tune, then eventually, you will come into harmony with the singer next to you.

- If you are walking alongside a strong walker, you will almost certainly liven to their pace.

- Put a good player on the football pitch, just as the game is flagging, and the whole tone can pick up.

This is the harmonic principle at work – and this is the unique way Alexander discovered to change the way of being, from tension to openness.

THINKING TOGETHER

Alexander recognised the significance of the mind/body relationship, and he was able to use it in his teaching. He asked his pupil to think with him.

- Firstly, the pupil needs to notice, to observe, the habit that causes harm – for example, crunching the neck as the head is pulled back and down.

- Secondly, the pupil needs to pause, to inhibit, in order to give time for the directions for the primary control to take place:
  "Let the neck be free so that the head can go forward and up".

And with this, the quality of non-doing, of effortlessness, has time to come into being.

- Thirdly, the movement must be co-ordinated. So when the pupil goes from standing to sitting, for example, the

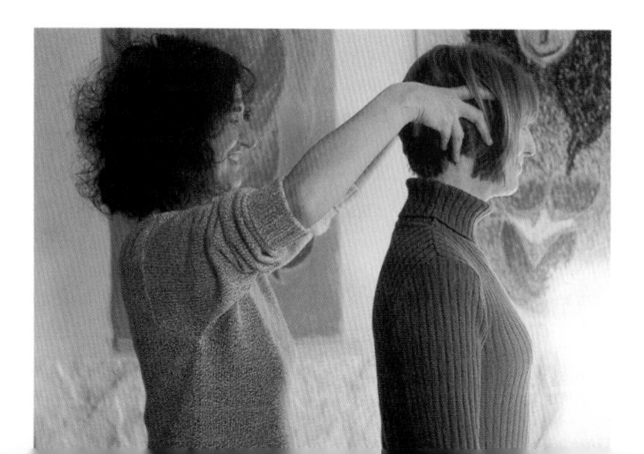

◄ *The same directions for primary control are given when the pupil is standing.*

movement coincides with the flow of directions, on strong, radiant, positive thinking.

This gives the movement the quality of flow, of non-doing, of effortlessness.

LEADING FROM WITHIN

By being the environment that he wished his students themselves to become, both in mind and body, Alexander was leading from within.

Unlike an army general pointing and shouting at his troops to go forward, Alexander was behaving more like a fire-man, leading his men into the fire from the front. Being there first.

Alexander did this with his hands on the pupil, and with his voice giving instructions. The pupil's body sensed what the thinking was by experience, and heard what the body should be thinking, by listening to Alexander's voice. This would all be done in the simple vocabulary of everyday use.

A typical session would be as follows:

- The pupil lies down on the table, and learns about the

directions for the primary control in relative stillness, having the limbs moved while the back remains resting on the table.

- Coming off the table, the same directions for the primary control are given, but now when standing and walking, then sitting in a chair, and standing up out of the chair.

- Many teachers now include squatting and crawling, and even rolling, in the vocabulary of movement. Anything is possible, once the primary control has been applied.

THE WIDER APPLICATION

If the principles of the Alexander Technique are involved, the applications are almost limitless. Musicians bring their instruments to their Alexander lessons, actors bring their speeches, singers bring their songs. All can be applied to the proper use of the self through the primary control.

Alexander teachers go to the riding schools to help riders

apply the work on horseback, they go to the sports field to help athletes, and to the swimming pool to teach swimmers to apply the primary control to their strokes. The scope is enormous.

In the end, the relationship of thinking together leads the pupil towards independence from the teacher. In time, the pupil learns to monitor himself, both in everyday activities and in the performance of their choice.

▶ *The directions are repeated when the pupil is sitting.*

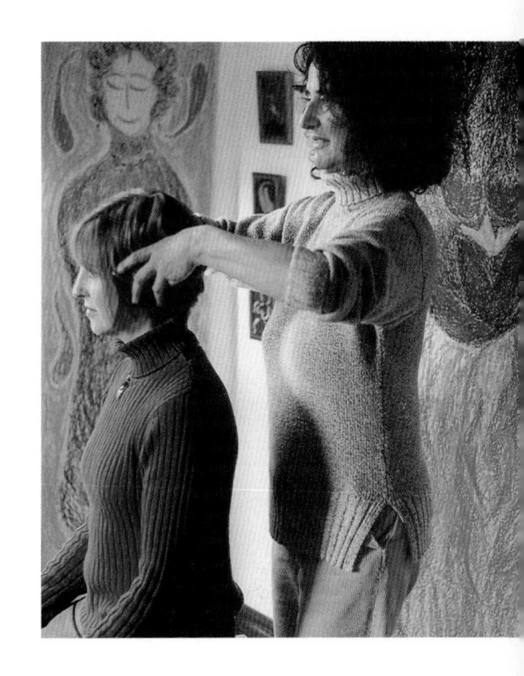

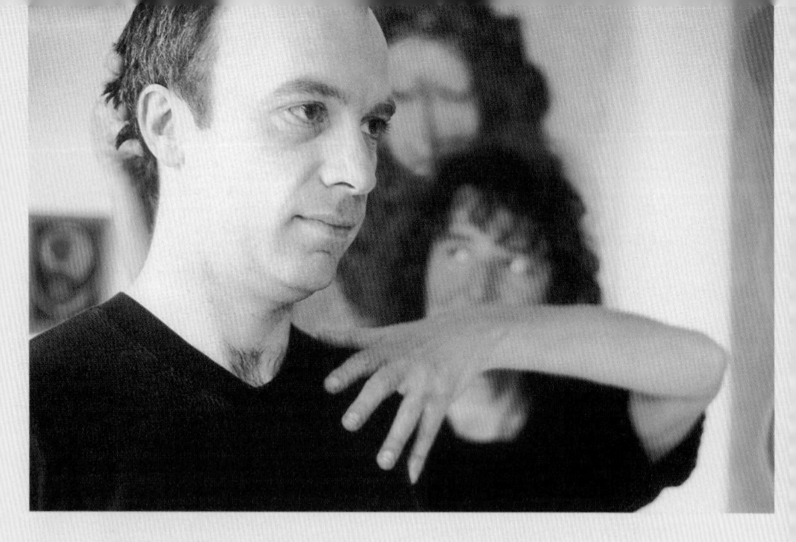

6 Will The Alexander Technique Work For Me?

Because Alexander worked on a vast number of different cases, ranging from professional actors to so-called incurables, there is obviously a large number of people who will find the therapy beneficial.

Drawing from my own personal experience, I would say there are three main categories of the type of situation it can help.

STRUCTURAL CONDITIONS

This category includes those with difficulties concerning the structure of the body itself.

For example, I came to the Alexander Technique because of a frozen shoulder. In time, I learned to think with my shoulder, both to keep it open and to prevent it from closing again.

I was taught how to think, both generally into the body, and specifically to the shoulder.

In the same category, I would include the following:

- Those with a permanently slumped upper back.

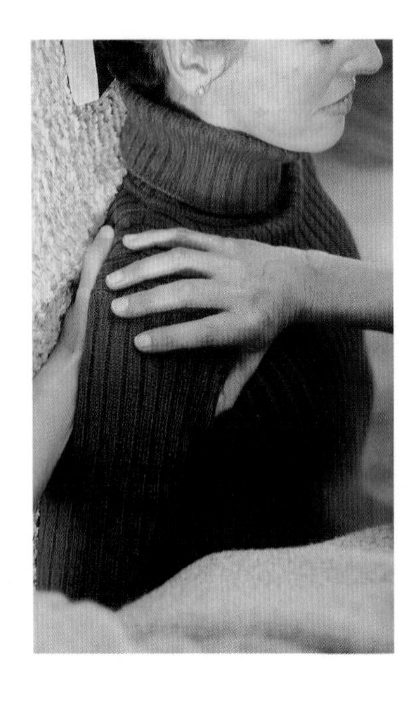

- The crunched neck of the dowager's hump.
- The fixed or stuck lower back.
- The clamped-in hips.
- The collapsed chest.

People with permanently fixed and painful states of structure benefit by learning to observe themselves. They discover how they got into the situation in the first place, and then how to think themselves out of that particularly tight corner.

◀ *Opening the shoulder: Chronic structural conditions, such as a frozen shoulder, will benefit from the Alexander Technique.*

This is achieved by learning a system that teaches the whole structure to stay open and out of compression.

NERVOUS CONDITIONS

This category includes people suffering from conditions related to the nervous system, such as migraines, asthma, general tension, anxiety and depression.

The individual is helped by learning a system that deals with the essential core of the being, and trains the mind to stay with the core and come away from the peripheries.

Learning to pause, to wait, to stop and think: "how am I going to approach this, from my structural centre, from my primary control, from my spine?", can have an enormously calming effect.

HIGH PERFORMANCE

This category includes runners, dancers, musicians, actors and singers, who are called on to perform at a high level of excellence.

These people can be helped by learning how to get the very, very best they can out of the

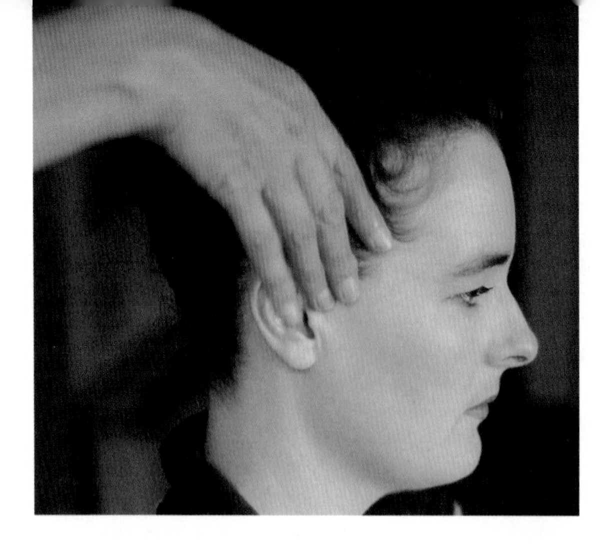

◀ *People who suffer from migraines, and stress-related conditions can often be helped.*

body when it us under the high demand of a refined and particular activity.

It is also very beneficial to learn both how to prepare the mind/body for a performance, and then how to wind down afterwards.

WHAT WILL I LEARN?

Pupils from all three categories will learn, both in principle and practice, how to apply the primary control to themselves, and the directions to use to achieve this.

With the help of a teacher's hands and voice, a student will learn these practices while sitting, standing and walking.

Perhaps of greatest interest, each pupil will learn that what they thought was 'natural' to them is, in fact, not natural, objectively, to the structure.

For instance, a student may think he is standing upright (and believes he has done so all of his life), but he may, in fact, be slanting backwards.

Alexander called this false impression of correctness that we all have 'faulty sensory awareness' or 'debauched kinaesthesia'.

In some cases, students learn where their bones are, and are able to sense them in movement. Often, a student comes to a lesson not knowing where their hip socket is, or how wide their collar bones actually are.

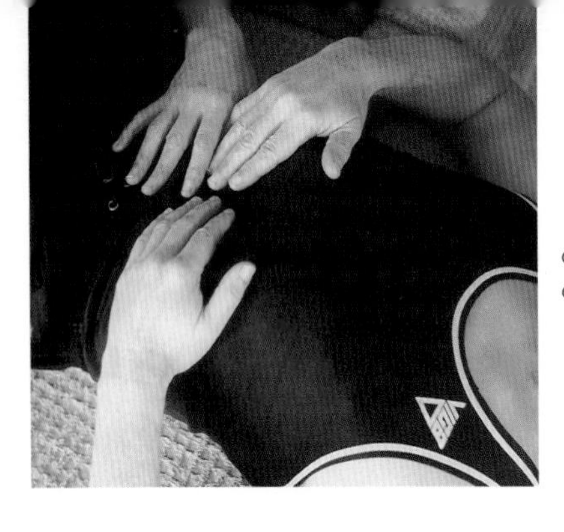

◀ *Back dropping to widen and open: Every pupil learns at their own pace.*

Acquiring his type of knowledge and awareness helps the pupil to benefit more completely from the therapy.

Finally, the student can expect, to some degree, to become his own teacher. The aim is for the student to learn to observe himself in daily life, and to apply the practice of the primary control to himself when the teacher is not there.

HOW LONG WILL IT TAKE?

Pupils often ask how many lessons are needed, and how

long will it take to benefit from the Alexander Technique.

This is difficult to answer – it is the same as asking how long it will take to master the cello or to learn German. My answer to a prospective pupil is this: it depends on how much you are willing to work on yourself, by yourself, at home.

It also depends on your background. If someone has already been involved with mind/body work, such as meditation, yoga or tai chi, they will often find the work easier than someone who has no such background.

Finally, it depends on how deeply entrenched your particular problem is. All these are variables.

Having made these points, I would estimate that a course would include from ten to twenty lessons on a once-weekly basis. This would progress on to once a fortnight, then once every three weeks or four weeks. A maintenance programme of once a month is ideal, once the initial stages of learning the technique and applying it in daily life have been accomplished.

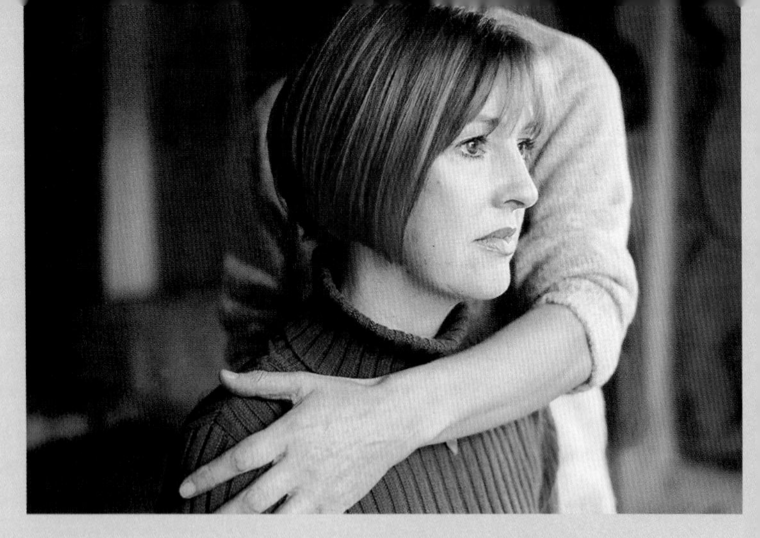

7 Three Great Benefits

We have examined the principles of the Alexander Technique, and we have looked at those who can be helped. However, there are three major universal benefits that should be considered.

PAIN MANAGEMENT

Research into pain management is being pioneered by a number of Alexander teachers, looking specifically at hospital patients.

However, many people encounter pain and discomfort in their everyday lives, and they have come to the Alexander Technique for help. As these people learn the principle of the primary control in their Alexander lessons, they are gradually able to make use of this system in their daily lives.

For example, a person may be sitting at their desk or at their computer, suffering from headaches and a cramped neck.

By self-observation, that individual will be able so see how he is misusing himself at work. He may notice that he is pulling his head back and down, and cramping his neck,

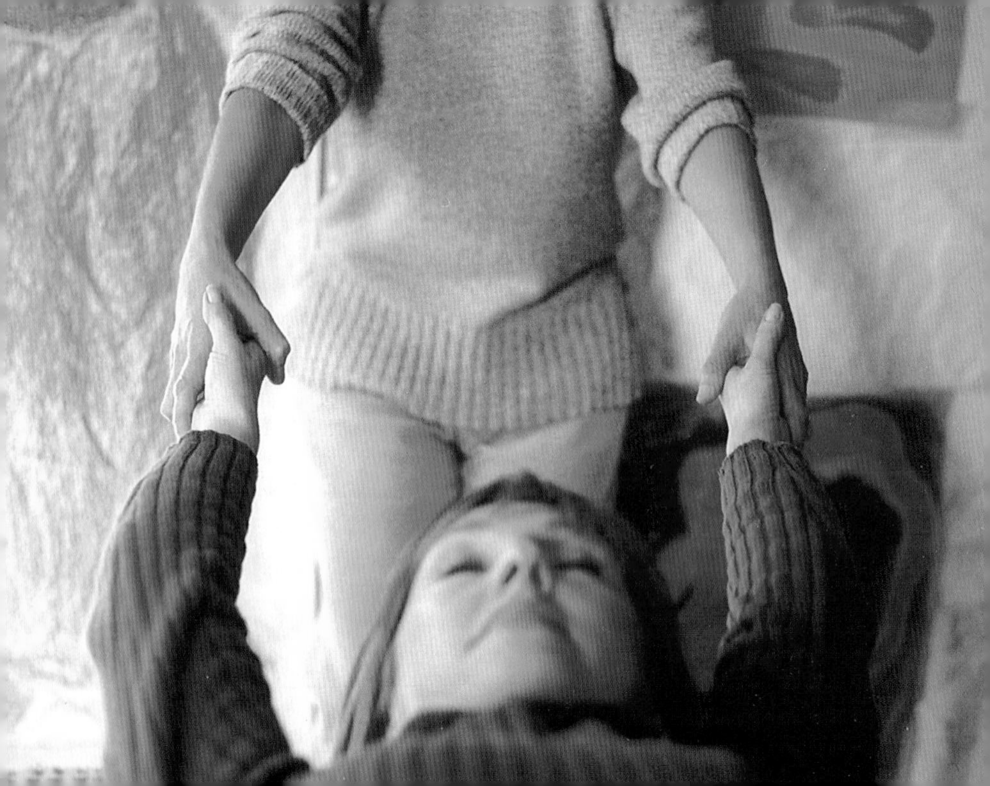

while he is working at his computer.

With the experience of Alexander lessons, he may be able to correct this misuse, simply by knowing how to free his neck and send his head forward and up, while still at the computer, without having to leave the job.

A simple correction like this, done many times through the day, can have the result of relieving pain. It is simple and fast to be able to correct yourself – and it is possible to do this through learning the Alexander Technique.

Eventually, a person will be able to see the trouble coming before it actually sets in. This is a skilful way of using the system of the Alexander Technique to prevent pain.

Likewise, a person with lower back pain may learn, through the Alexander Technique, to think into his back in such a way as to release it, while still sitting at his desk.

A violinist, having studied the

◀ *Opposite: The Alexander Technique has helped with the relief and management of pain.*

Alexander Technique, may be able to notice how she is misusing the shoulder while bowing.

When uncorrected, it causes her considerable pain, but now it can be corrected while still playing. It is very skilful to be able to do this while in the process of playing, but with lessons and time, it is highly possible.

In this way, the Alexander Technique, once properly mastered, becomes a tool for skilful interception. It can prevent pain setting in, and the individual is empowered to change the situation, of being able to choose their response to the activity.

FINDING PLEASURE

The second benefit of studying the Alexander Technique is the person's ability to 'pause' – referred to as 'inhibition'. Between stimulus and response there is a gap, a pause, into which a person can make a choice with their conscious mind.

For instance, if you are taking a walk in the country, you may give yourself permission to

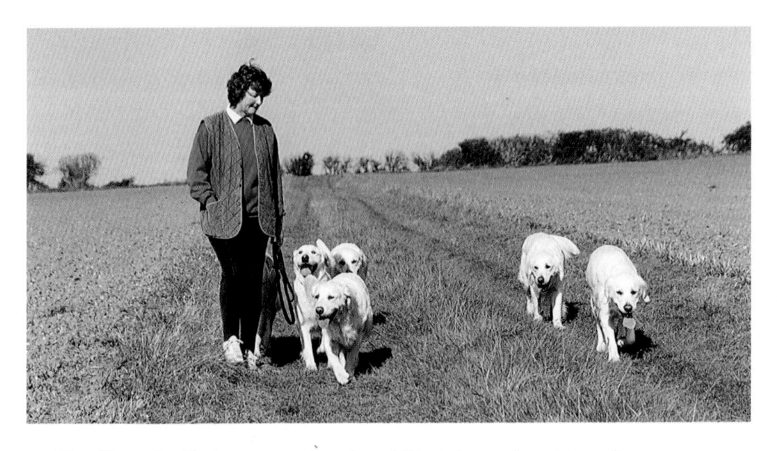

▲ *The Alexander Technique teaches the ability to 'pause' and to make a controlled decision.*

pause at a fork in the path and ask yourself: "Where do I really want to go – into the shade of the woods, or into the open sunlit space of the hills?"

When you started walking, it

was raining, so the woods seemed like the right path to take. Now the rain has stopped, the whole situation is different.

This is the moment to pause, and ask yourself: "What do I really want to do?" You have the power to choose because you caught the moment in time – and this can give a sudden increase in joy, quite unexpectedly.

In the same way, the person who is dieting, confronted with a large and tempting buffet, may find that, with the ability to pause and to return to the primary control, they can stop to ask "Do I really want this Death By Chocolate cake, or would my digestion prefer a milky coffee?" There is a choice; I am in charge of the situation, and that, in itself, gives a sense of empowerment.

And finally, during sex, the ability to pause and return to the primary control, will stop the rush, to choose this embrace instead of that, to wait, to do it differently, to prolong the pleasure. After all, you are the centre of your own activities.

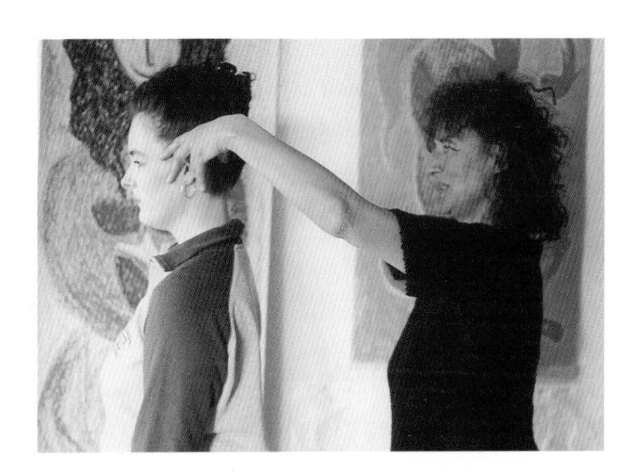

▶ *Let the 'up', take you up.*

THE RADIANT WAY

The third benefit of learning the Alexander Technique is that it deals not only with gravity, the earth, but also with anti-gravity, with radiance, with the sun. The word used for this in the Alexander Technique is 'up'.

As we know, all of nature is

affected by the sun, by anti-gravity, as it grows upwards. All we are doing in the Alexander Technique is simply joining in, taking a principle of nature and bringing it to our conscious awareness.

So if you are walking along a country lane, you can be aware of your feet and their deep connection to the earth. You can also be aware of the uplift of the sunlight, and, just by paying attention, you can sense the forces of radiance lifting you gently out of your hips, out of your ankles, and helping your spirits lift up into the light, without effort or strain, but simply by being aware of the 'up'.

This has the benefit of giving us a sense of lightness, of ease, and of spaciousness in our joints. We can take pleasure in small things, and we are always empowered to make a choice.

How to find us...

The Alexander Technique is taught all over the world. It is taught privately by teachers who work from home, and by practitioners who work in alternative clinics for complementary medicine, along with osteopaths, homoeopaths, acupuncturists, etc.

The Society of Teachers for the Alexander Technique (STAT):
129, Camden Mews,
London, NW1 9AH.
Telephone: 0207 284 3338.
www.stat.org.uk

USEFUL WEBSITES

www.alexandertechnique.com
www.alexandertechnique.com/atonline
www.Alexander-Technique.org.uk
www.lpb.com/alex/
www.ati-net.com

About the author

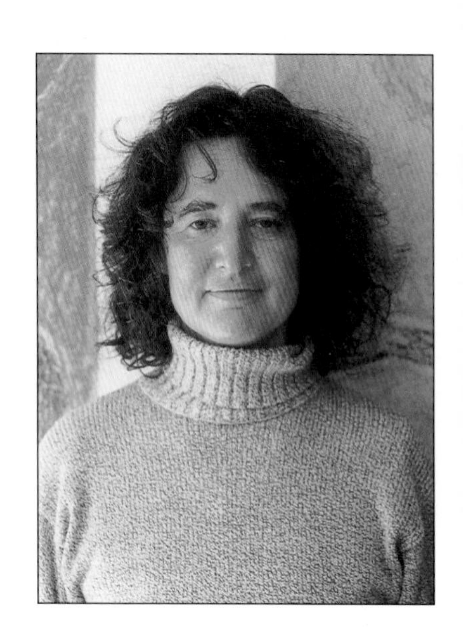

Joan Diamond lives and works in Kendal, in the Lake District. She has a private practice at home and she trains teachers at the Fellside Centre in Kendal. She has been devoted to the teaching and study of the Alexander Technique for 16 years.

Other titles in the series

- Understanding Acupressure
- Understanding Acupuncture
- Understanding Aromatherapy
- Understanding Echinacea
- Understanding Evening Primrose
- Understanding Feng Shui
- Understanding Fish Oils
- Understanding Flower Remedies
- Understanding Garlic
- Understanding Head Massage
- Understanding Kinesiology
- Understanding Lavender
- Understanding Pilates
- Understanding Reflexology
- Understanding Reiki
- Understanding Shiatsu
- Understanding St. John's Wort
- Understanding Yoga

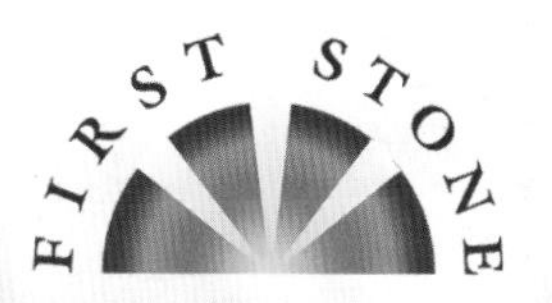

Photography: Russell Colman.
Models: Neil Malone, Paul Baxter, Monica O' Dare and Joanne O' Callaghan – all students of the Cumbria Alexander School.

First published 2003 by First Stone Publishing
4/5 The Marina, Harbour Road, Lydney, Gloucestershire, GL15 5ET

ISBN 1-904439-004

Printed and bound in Hong Kong through Printworks International Ltd.